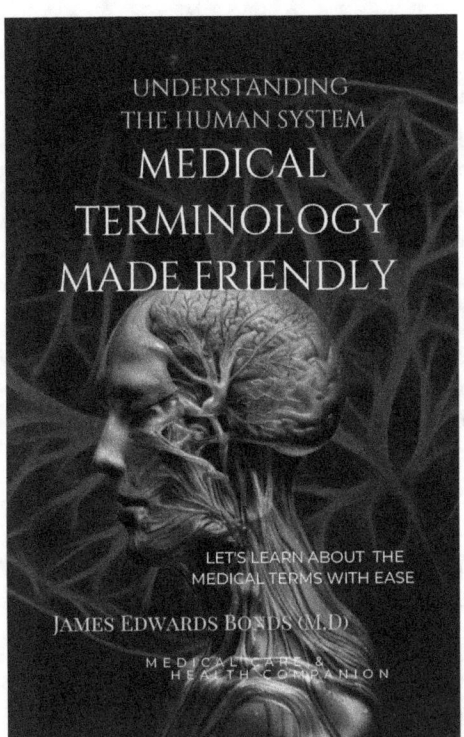

UNDERSTANDING
THE HUMAN SYSTEM

MEDICAL
TERMINOLOGY
MADE FRIENDLY

LET'S LEARN ABOUT THE
MEDICAL TERMS WITH EASE

JAMES EDWARDS BONDS (M.D)

MEDICAL CARE &
HEALTH COMPANION

About the Author

I am really thrilled that you have decided to take a keen interest in Medical Terminologies. I am **Dr. James Edwards Bonds (M.D),** the brilliant mind behind "Medical Terminology Made Friendly,". I'm an accomplished healthcare professional with a passion for simplifying complex subjects. With years of experience, I've witnessed firsthand, how medical terminology can be a barrier for many individuals.

Fueled by a desire to bridge this knowledge gap, I decided to embark on a mission to make medical terminology accessible to all. I have a soft spot, really for unique intricate medical concepts and transforming them into relatable, easy-to-understand language. This skill has earned me recognition and respect within the healthcare community.

If complex medical terms and jargon leave you feeling like you're navigating a foreign language? Don't be scared! "Medical Terminology Made Friendly" carefully explains the world of healthcare terminology and makes it accessible to everyone, whether you're a medical professional, a student, or simply a curious individual. Inside the pages of this eBook, you'll find:

- A user-friendly guide to the building blocks of medical terminology.
- Engaging explanations and relatable examples that ensure you grasp concepts quickly and easily.
- Essential terminology for various medical specialties, from anatomy to pharmacology.
- Tips and abbreviations tricks for remembering challenging medical terms. Real-world applications, making the content relevant and memorable.

"Medical Terminology Made Friendly" is your trusted companion on the path to understanding and mastering medical language. Whether you're studying for a healthcare profession, preparing for medical exams, or simply eager to enhance your medical literacy, this book will transform the daunting into the doable. Say goodbye to the intimidation factor, and embrace the world of healthcare terminology with confidence and a friendly smile. Start your journey today!

Dr. James Edwards Bonds (M.D)

Medical Terminology Made Friendly: Understanding The Human Body Systems

Table of Contents

Understanding the Importance of Medical Terminology

Medical terminology is the language of healthcare. It serves as a common foundation for healthcare professionals, enabling effective communication, accurate documentation, and improved patient care. In this introductory chapter, we explore the significance of medical terminology in the following sections:

The Language of Medicine: An overview of how medical terminology is a specialized language that simplifies complex medical concepts.

Precision and Clarity: How precise terminology reduces ambiguity and ensures clear communication among healthcare providers.

Global Application: The international use of medical terminology and its role in facilitating communication across borders.

Career Advancement: How a strong grasp of medical terminology can enhance career opportunities in healthcare.

Chapter Summary: A brief recap of the key points discussed in this chapter.

Throughout this ebook, we will delve deeper into the components and applications of medical terminology, providing you with the knowledge and tools to navigate the intricate world of healthcare language.

How to Use This Book
This section provides guidance on how to effectively utilize this ebook for learning and reference. Here's what you can expect in this part:

1. Navigating the Chapters: Instructions on how the ebook is structured, including the table of contents and chapter organization.

2. Learning Approach: Tips on how to best absorb and retain medical terminology, including the use of examples, practice exercises, and self-assessment.

3. Key Features: An overview of any special features, such as case studies, glossary, or online resources, that enhance your learning experience.

4. Note-Taking and Annotations: Recommendations for taking notes, highlighting important information, and customizing this ebook for your personal needs.

5. Interactive Learning: If this ebook includes online resources or interactive elements, we'll guide you on how to access and use them.

6. Getting Help: Contact information or support resources for any questions or issues related to the ebook.

By understanding how to navigate and engage with this ebook, you can make the most of the valuable content and resources it offers for learning and mastering medical terminology.

We will explore the fundamental components of medical terminology that will provide you with a strong starting point for understanding the language of healthcare. An overview of what you'll find in this chapter:

Word Roots, Prefixes, and Suffixes
- Definition and importance of word elements in medical terms.
- Exploring common word roots, prefixes, and suffixes.
- How to combine these elements to create medical terms.

- Building and Decoding Medical Terms**
- The structure of medical terms: combining roots, prefixes, and suffixes.
- Tips and techniques for dissecting complex medical words.
- Practice exercises for building and decoding medical terms.

Common Medical Abbreviations

- A list of frequently used medical abbreviations and their meanings.
- Understanding the importance of abbreviations in healthcare documentation.
- Cautions and guidelines for using medical abbreviations safely.

Building and Decoding Medical Terms

In this section, we dive deeper into the structure of medical terms and provide you with the skills to construct and decipher these terms effectively. Here's what you'll learn:

Anatomy of a Medical Term: A breakdown of a medical term into its constituent parts, including root words, prefixes, and suffixes.

Combining Elements: Guidelines on how to combine these word elements to form meaningful medical terms.

Decoding Medical Terms: Step-by-step strategies to interpret complex medical terms by recognizing their components.

Practice Exercises: Interactive exercises and examples to reinforce your ability to build and decode medical terms.

By the end of this section, you'll have a solid understanding of how medical terms are structured and the ability to dissect and understand a wide range of medical vocabulary. This knowledge is essential for communication within the healthcare field and will be invaluable throughout your medical terminology learning journey.

Common Medical Abbreviations

These are some of the common medical abbreviations:

1. Rx: Prescription

2. Dx: Diagnosis

3. Tx : Treatment

4. Hx : Medical history

5. CC: Chief Complaint

6. CXR: Chest X-ray

7. ECG or EKG: Electrocardiogram

8. MRI: Magnetic Resonance Imaging

9. CT: Computed Tomography

10. BP: Blood Pressure

11. HR: Heart Rate

12. RR: Respiratory Rate
13. TPR: Temperature, Pulse, Respiration

14. CBC: Complete Blood Count

15. WBC: White Blood Cell

16. RBC: Red Blood Cell

17. ESR: Erythrocyte
Sedimentation Rate

18. IV: Intravenous

19. PO: By mouth (oral)

20. NPO: Nothing by mouth (nothing per oral)

21. PRN: As needed (pro re nata)

22. QD: Once a day (every day)

23. BID: Twice a day (two times a day)

24. TID: Three times a day (three times a day

25. QID: Four times a day (four times a day)

26. QHS: Every night at bedtime

27. NKA: No Known Allergies

28. SOB: Shortness of Breath

29. GI: Gastrointestinal

30. GU: Genitourinary

31. CVA: Cerebrovascular Accident (Stroke)

32. MI: Myocardial Infarction (Heart Attack)

33. COPD: Chronic Obstructive Pulmonary Disease

34. GERD: Gastroesophageal Reflux Disease

35. DM: Diabetes Mellitus

36. HTN: Hypertension (High Blood Pressure)

37. CA: Cancer

38. MMS: Multiple Sclerosis

39. HIV: Human Immunodeficiency Virus

40. AIDS: Acquired Immunodeficiency Syndrome

41. UTI: Urinary Tract Infection

42. OB/GYN: Obstetrics and Gynecology

43. ENT: Ear, Nose, and Throat

44. ASAP: As Soon As Possible

45. N/V: Nausea and Vomiting

46. CABG: Coronary Artery Bypass Graft

47. CHF: Congestive Heart Failure

48. SIRS: Systemic Inflammatory Response Syndrome

49. PT: Physical Therapy

50. OT: Occupational Therapy

51. ROM: Range of Motion

52. POA: Power of Attorney

53. DOA: Dead on Arrival

54. NPO: Nil per os (Nothing by mouth)

55. DC: Discharge

56. ROS: Review of Systems

57. LOC: Loss of Consciousness

58. Fx: Fracture

59. VS: Vital Signs

60. DNR: Do Not Resuscitate

61. ICU: Intensive Care Unit

62. ER: Emergency Room

63. NICU: Neonatal Intensive Care Unit

64. OB: Obstetrics

65. PPD: Purified Protein Derivative (Tuberculosis skin test)

66. DVT: Deep Vein Thrombosis

67. ABG: Arterial Blood Gas

68. CPR: Cardiopulmonary Resuscitation

69. APAP: Acetaminophen (Paracetamol)

70. GER: Gastroesophageal Reflux

71. PPI: Proton Pump Inhibitor

72. DMARD: Disease-Modifying Antirheumatic Drug

73. TSH: Thyroid-Stimulating Hormone

74. ICD: International Classification of Diseases

75. MRI: Magnetic
Resonance Imaging

76. TPA: Tissue Plasminogen Activator

77. IVF: In Vitro Fertilization

78. ENT: Ear, Nose, and Throat

79. PID: Pelvic Inflammatory

80. ARDS: Acute Respiratory Distress Syndrome

Please note that this list includes a variety of medical abbreviations commonly used in healthcare and medical documentation.

Human Body Terminologies

1. Anatomy: The study of the structure and organization of the body.

2. Physiology: The study of how the body's systems and organs function.

3. Organ System: A group of organs that work together to perform specific functions (e.g., the circulatory system).

4. Tissue: A group of cells that have a similar structure and function.

5. Organ: A structure composed of multiple tissues that performs a specific function (e.g., the heart).

6. Cell: The basic unit of life and the smallest functional unit in the body.

7. Nervous System: The body's network of nerves and cells that transmit signals.

8. Circulatory System: The system responsible for transporting blood, oxygen, and nutrients throughout the body.

9. Respiratory System: The system responsible for breathing and gas exchange.

10. Digestive System: The system responsible for breaking down food and absorbing nutrients.

11. Muscular System: The system responsible for movement and supporting the body.

12. Skeletal System: The system of bones and cartilage that provides support and protection.

13. Endocrine System: The system of glands that produce hormones.

14. Reproductive System: The system responsible for human reproduction.

15. Integumentary System: The skin and associated structures that protect the body.

16. Immune System: The body's defense against infection and disease.

17. Lymphatic System: A network of vessels and organs that help transport lymph and fight infections.

18. Urinary System: The system responsible for filtering and excreting waste products from the body.

19. Homeostasis: The body's ability to maintain a stable internal environment.

20. Metabolism: The chemical processes that occur within the body to maintain life.

21. Neuron: A nerve cell, the basic building block of the nervous system.

22. Artery: Blood vessels that carry oxygenated blood away from the heart.

23. Vein: Blood vessels that carry deoxygenated blood back to the heart.

24. Capillary: Tiny blood vessels that allow for the exchange of nutrients and gases between blood and tissues.

25. Cardiovascular: Relating to the heart and blood vessels.

26. Dermatology: The branch of medicine related to the skin.

27. Orthopedics: The branch of medicine dealing with the musculoskeletal system.

28. Ophthalmology: The branch of medicine related to the eyes.

29. Gynecology: The branch of medicine focused on female reproductive health.

30. Urology: The branch of medicine concerned with the urinary system.

31. Pediatrics: The branch of medicine specializing in children's healthcare.

32. Geriatrics: The branch of medicine focusing on elderly patients.

33. Physiotherapy: The treatment of physical dysfunction or injury through exercise and physical methods.

34. Neurology: The branch of medicine concerned with the nervous system.

35. Gastroenterology: The branch of medicine specializing in the digestive system.

36. Endocrinology: The branch of medicine dealing with the endocrine system and hormones.

37. Pulmonology: The branch of medicine focused on respiratory health.

38. Hematology: The study of blood and blood disorders.

39. Oncology: The branch of medicine dealing with cancer.

40. Rheumatology: The study of disorders affecting the joints and connective tissues.

These are some fundamental terms related to the human body and its various systems and functions.

Anatomical Regions and Body System Terminologies

These are the Terminologies related to anatomical regions:

Anatomical Regions

1. Anterior: The front or forward part of the body.

2. Posterior: The rear or back part of the body.

3. Superior: Above or closer to the head.

4. Inferior: Below or closer to the feet.

5. Proximal: Nearer to the point of attachment or origin.

6. Distal: Farther from the point of attachment or origin.

7. Medial: Closer to the midline of the body.

8. Lateral: Farther from the midline of the body.

9. Cranial:Pertaining to the skull.
10. Caudal: Toward the tailbone (coccyx).

11. Superficial: Closer to the surface of the body.

12. Deep: Farther from the surface, more internal.

13. Peripheral: Away from the center or core.

14. Bilateral: Present on both sides of the body.

15. Unilateral: Present on only one side of the body.

16. Dorsal: Relating to the back of the body.

17. Ventral: Referring to the front of the body.

Body Systems Terminologies

1. Integumentary System: The skin and its associated structures, providing protection and regulating temperature.

2. Nervous System: The network of nerves and cells that transmit signals, controlling bodily functions.

3. Circulatory System: Responsible for blood circulation and nutrient transport.

4. Respiratory System: Facilitates breathing and gas exchange in the lungs.

5. Digestive System: Processes food and absorbs nutrients.

6. Muscular System: Enables movement and supports the body.

7. Skeletal System: Composed of bones and cartilage, providing support and protection.

8. Endocrine System: Composed of glands that produce and secrete hormones.

9. Reproductive System: Involved in human reproduction.

10. Lymphatic System: A network of vessels and organs responsible for immune function.

11. Urinary System: Filters and excretes waste products from the body.

12. Homeostasis: The body's ability to maintain a stable internal environment.

13. Metabolism: The chemical processes within the body that sustain life.

These terminologies help describe the location, orientation, and organization of anatomical structures and the major systems that make up the human body.

Organs, Tissues, and Cells Terminologies

Organs Terminologies:

1. Heart: The muscular organ responsible for pumping blood throughout the circulatory system.

2. Lungs: The primary organs for respiration and gas exchange.

3. Brain: The central organ of the nervous system, responsible for cognition and control of bodily functions.

4. Liver: A vital organ involved in metabolic processes, detoxification, and nutrient storage.

5. Kidneys: Organs that filter waste and excess substances from the blood.
6. Stomach: A digestive organ responsible for breaking down food.

7. Intestines: The digestive organs where nutrient absorption occurs.

8. Pancreas: An organ that produces digestive enzymes and regulates blood sugar.

9. Spleen: Involved in blood filtration and the immune system.

10. Gallbladder: Stores bile produced by the liver for digestion.

11. Bladder: The organ responsible for storing and expelling urine.

12. Uterus: The female reproductive organ where a fetus develops.

13. Ovaries: Female reproductive organs that produce eggs and hormones.

14. Testes: Male reproductive organs responsible for sperm production.

15. Thyroid: A gland that regulates metabolism.

16. Adrenal Glands:.Glands involved in stress response and hormone production.

17. Lymph Nodes: Small structures that filter lymph and participate in immune responses.

18. Skin: The body's largest organ, serving as a protective barrier.

19. Bone: The rigid organ providing support and protection.

20. Muscles: Organs responsible for movement and support.

Tissues Terminologies:

1. Epithelial Tissue: The tissue that covers body surfaces, lines cavities, and forms glands.

2. Connective Tissue: Provides support and connects various body structures.

3. Muscle Tissue: Enables movement and contraction.

4. Nervous Tissue: Transmits electrical impulses and coordinates bodily functions.

Cells Terminologies:

1. Cell Membrane: The outer layer of a cell, regulating the passage of substances in and out.

2. Nucleus: The cell's control center, containing genetic material (DNA).

3. Cytoplasm: The fluid within the cell, where various organelles are found.

4. Mitochondria: Organelles that produce energy (ATP) for the cell.

5. Endoplasmic Reticulum (ER): Involved in protein and lipid synthesis.

6. Ribosomes: Structures responsible for protein synthesis.

7. Golgi Apparatus: Modifies, packages, and transports proteins and lipids.

8. Lysosomes: Contain enzymes for cellular digestion.

9. Cytoskeleton: Provides structure and support to the cell.

10. Cell Nucleolus: Involved in the production of ribosomes.

These terminologies describe various organs, tissues, and cellular components in the human body, highlighting their functions and roles in maintaining overall health and homeostasis.

Medical Terms for Body Movements and Positions Terminologies

Body Movements Terminologies:

1. Flexion: Bending a joint to decrease the angle between two bones.

2. Extension: Straightening a joint to increase the angle between two bones.

3. Abduction: Moving a body part away from the midline of the body.

4. Adduction: Moving a body part toward the midline of the body.

5. Rotation: Turning a bone around its own axis.

6. Circumduction: Moving a body part in a circular path.

7. Elevation: Raising or lifting a body part.

8. Depression: Lowering a body part.

9. Pronation: Turning the palm of the hand downward.

10. Supination: Turning the palm of the hand upward.

11. Dorsiflexion: Bending the foot upward at the ankle.

12. Plantarflexion: Pointing the foot downward at the ankle.

13. Inversion: Turning the sole of the foot inward.

14. Eversion: Turning the sole of the foot outward.

15. Protraction: Moving a body part forward.

16. Retraction: Moving a body part backward.

17. Opposition: Bringing the thumb and another finger together.

Body Positions and Planes Terminologies:

18. Prone: Lying face down.
19. Supine: Lying face up.

20. Lateral: Lying on the side.

21. Medial: Toward the midline of the body.

22. Superior: Positioned above another structure.
23. Inferior: Positioned below another structure.

24. Anterior (Ventral): Toward the front of the body.

25. Posterior (Dorsal): Toward the back of the body.

26. Proximal: Nearer to the point of attachment or origin.

27. Distal: Farther from the point of attachment or origin.

28. Supine: Lying face up.

29. Prone: Lying face down.

30. Fowler's Position: Sitting with the upper body elevated.

31. Lithotomy Position: Lying on the back with knees and hips flexed and thighs abducted and rotated externally.

Medical terms related to diseases and diagnosis:

Disease and Condition Terminologies:

1. Disease: An abnormal condition that impairs normal bodily functioning.

2. Disorder: A disruption of normal bodily structure or function.

3. Syndrome: A set of symptoms that occur together and characterize a particular condition.

4. Pathology: The study of disease and its causes.

5. Etiology: The cause or origin of a disease.

6. Symptom: A subjective indication of a disease or condition experienced by the patient.

7. Sign: An objective, observable indication of a disease or condition.

8. Diagnosis: The identification of a disease or condition through examination and testing.

9. Prognosis: The expected course and outcome of a disease or condition.

10. Remission: A period when the signs and symptoms of a disease decrease or disappear.

11. Chronic: Persisting over an extended period, often referring to long-term diseases.

12. Acute: Having a rapid onset and a short course, often referring to short-term illnesses.

13. Hereditary: Passed down from one generation to the next.

14. Congenital: Present at birth, often referring to birth defects.

15. Idiopathic: Of unknown cause.

16. Autoimmune: Conditions where the immune system attacks the body's own tissues.

17. Infection: Invasion and multiplication of microorganisms in the body.

18. Contagious: Capable of spreading from person to person.

19. Endemic: Common or native to a specific geographic area.

20. Epidemic: A sudden increase in the number of cases of a disease in a community.

21. Pandemic: An epidemic that spreads across a large geographic area.

22. Outbreak: A localized increase in the incidence of a disease.

23. Quarantine: Isolation to prevent the spread of disease.

24. Vaccine: A substance used to stimulate the immune system to prevent disease.

25. Antibiotic: A medication used to treat bacterial infections.

Diagnosis and Testing Terminologies:

26. Physical Examination: A visual and manual inspection of a patient's body.

27. Medical History: Information about a patient's past and present health.

28. Clinical Assessment: The evaluation of a patient's medical condition.

29. Laboratory Tests: Diagnostic tests performed on bodily fluids or tissues.

30. Radiology: The use of medical imaging techniques for diagnosis (e.g., X-rays, CT scans).

31. Biopsy: The removal and examination of a sample of tissue for diagnosis.

32. Ultrasound: High-frequency sound waves used for imaging internal structures.

33. MRI: Magnetic Resonance Imaging, a non-invasive imaging technique.

34. CT Scan: Computed Tomography, a specialized X-ray technique.

35. Colonoscopy: Examination of the colon using a flexible tube with a camera.

36. Endoscopy: Visual examination of internal structures using a flexible tube.

37. Blood Test: Analysis of blood to assess health and diagnose conditions.

38. Diagnosis Code: A standardized code used for medical billing and insurance purposes.

39. Screening: Testing or examination for the early detection of a disease.

40. Biological Marker (Biomarker): A measurable indicator of a biological condition.

These terms help healthcare professionals describe, diagnose, and understand various diseases and conditions, as well as the processes involved in making medical diagnoses.

Medical Imaging and Terminology

Below are some of the medical terms related to medical imaging and diagnostic procedures:

Medical Imaging Terminologies:

1. Radiography: The use of X-rays to produce images of the inside of the body.

2. X-ray: A form of electromagnetic radiation used for imaging bones and tissues.

3. Computed Tomography (CT): A diagnostic imaging procedure that uses X-rays to create detailed cross-sectional images of the body.

4. Magnetic Resonance Imaging (MRI): A non-invasive imaging technique that uses magnetic fields and radio waves to create detailed images of the body's structures.

5. Ultrasound: A diagnostic imaging technique that uses high-frequency sound waves to produce images of internal organs and tissues.

6. Nuclear Medicine: A branch of medical imaging that uses radioactive substances to examine organ function and structure.

7. Positron Emission Tomography (PET): A nuclear medicine imaging technique that assesses metabolic activity in the body.

8. Mammography: An X-ray technique for breast imaging used in breast cancer screening.

9. Fluoroscopy: A real-time X-ray technique used for visualizing moving internal structures.

10. Angiography: A diagnostic procedure that uses contrast dye and X-rays to visualize blood vessels.

11. Doppler Ultrasound: A specialized ultrasound technique used to assess blood flow in vessels.

12. Bone Scan: A nuclear medicine procedure to detect abnormalities in bones.

13. Echocardiography: Ultrasound of the heart to assess its structure and function.

14. Magnetic Resonance Angiography (MRA): An MRI technique used to visualize blood vessels.

15. Myelography: An X-ray examination of the spinal cord and its surrounding structures.

16. Barium Enema: A contrast X-ray used to visualize the large intestine.

17. Endoscopy: A procedure that uses a flexible tube with a camera to view the inside of the body.

18. Arthroscopy: An endoscopic procedure to examine and treat joint conditions.

19. Cystoscopy: An endoscopic procedure to visualize the inside of the bladder.

20. Colonoscopy: Endoscopic examination of the colon and rectum.

21. Fluorodeoxyglucose (FDG): A radioactive glucose analog used in PET scans.

22. Gamma Camera: A device used in nuclear medicine to detect gamma radiation.

23. PACS (Picture Archiving and Communication System): A digital system for managing medical images.

24. Radiation Therapy: The use of high-energy radiation to treat diseases, including cancer.

25. DICOM (Digital Imaging and Communications in Medicine): A standard for transmitting and storing medical images.

The following are some medical terms related to procedures and treatments:

Medical Procedures

1. Surgery: The branch of medicine that involves cutting into the body for diagnosis, treatment, or repair.

2. Biopsy: The removal and examination of a sample of tissue for diagnostic purposes.

3. Endoscopy: The use of a flexible tube with a camera to visualize and diagnose internal structures.

4. Colonoscopy: An endoscopic examination of the colon and rectum.

5. Angioplasty: A procedure to open narrowed or blocked blood vessels, often used in coronary angioplasty.

6. Laparoscopy: Minimally invasive surgery using small incisions and a camera for visualization.

7. Arthroscopy: An endoscopic procedure to examine and treat joint conditions.

8. Cardiac Catheterization: A diagnostic procedure to examine the heart's blood vessels and chambers.

9. Hysterectomy: Surgical removal of the uterus.

10. Appendectomy: Surgical removal of the appendix.

11. Cholecystectomy: Surgical removal of the gallbladder.

12. Cesarean Section (C-Section): Surgical delivery of a baby through an incision in the mother's abdomen.

13. Electrocardiogram (ECG or EKG): A test that records the electrical activity of the heart.

14. Pulmonary Function Test (PFT): A test that measures lung function and capacity.

15. Bronchoscopy: An endoscopic procedure to examine the airways and lungs.

16. Bone Marrow Biopsy: A procedure to examine bone marrow for disorders.

17. Dialysis: A medical procedure for patients with kidney failure to remove waste products from the blood.

18. Radiotherapy: The use of high-energy radiation to treat diseases, including cancer.

19. Chemotherapy: Treatment of diseases, especially cancer, using chemical substances.

20. Physical Therapy (PT): A rehabilitative treatment to improve physical function and mobility.

21. Occupational Therapy (OT): Therapy to help individuals with physical or mental challenges regain daily life skills.

22. Speech Therapy: Treatment for speech and communication disorders.

23. Phlebotomy: The process of drawing blood for testing or donation.

24. Lumbar Puncture (Spinal Tap): A diagnostic procedure to collect cerebrospinal fluid for analysis.

25. MRI (Magnetic Resonance Imaging):A non-invasive imaging technique using magnetic fields and radio waves.

26. CT Scan (Computed Tomography): An X-ray technique used for detailed cross-sectional imaging.

27. Ultrasound: Imaging using high-frequency sound waves.

28. X-ray: A form of electromagnetic radiation used for imaging bones and tissues.

29. LVaccination: The administration of vaccines to prevent infectious diseases.

Treatments

30. Antibiotics: Medications used to treat bacterial infections.

31. Antivirals: Medications used to treat viral infections.

32. Antifungals: Medications used to treat fungal infections.

33. Anticoagulants: Medications that prevent blood clot formation.

34. Analgesics: Pain-relieving medications.

35. Chemotherapy: The use of drugs to treat cancer.

36. Immunotherapy: Treatment that stimulates or enhances the body's immune response.

37. Physical Therapy: Treatment to improve physical function and mobility.

38. Radiation Therapy: The use of radiation to treat diseases, especially cancer.

39. Psychological Counseling: Therapy for mental and emotional disorders.

40. Rehabilitation: A multidisciplinary approach to restore function after injury or illness.

41. Dietary Therapy: Nutrition-focused treatment for various medical conditions.

42. Hormone Replacement Therapy (HRT):Treatment to replace hormones that the body no longer produces in sufficient quantities.

These terms cover various medical procedures and treatment options used to diagnose, manage, and cure medical conditions and diseases.

Surgical Procedures and Instruments

Surgical Procedures

1. Appendectomy: Surgical removal of the appendix.

2. Cholecystectomy: Surgical removal of the gallbladder.

3. Hysterectomy: Surgical removal of the uterus.

4. Laparoscopy: Minimally invasive surgery using small incisions and a camera for visualization.

5. Arthroscopy: An endoscopic procedure to examine and treat joint conditions.

6. Colonoscopy: An endoscopic examination of the colon and rectum.

7. Cesarean Section (C-Section): Surgical delivery of a baby through an incision in the mother's abdomen.

8. Cardiac Bypass Surgery (CABG): A procedure to bypass blocked coronary arteries.

9. Laminectomy: Removal of the lamina of a vertebra to relieve spinal pressure.

10. Mastectomy: Surgical removal of the breast.

11. Thyroidectomy: Surgical removal of the thyroid gland.

12. Tonsillectomy: Surgical removal of the tonsils.

13. Hip Replacement (Hip Arthroplasty): Surgical procedure to replace a damaged hip joint with an artificial one.

14. Knee Replacement (Knee Arthroplasty): Surgical procedure to replace a damaged knee joint with an artificial one.

15. Gastric Bypass Surgery: Weight loss surgery that reduces the size of the stomach and bypasses part of the small intestine.

16. Corneal Transplant (Corneal Keratoplasty): Surgical procedure to replace a damaged cornea with a healthy one.

17. Thoracotomy: Surgical incision into the chest cavity.

18. Craniotomy: Surgical removal of a portion of the skull to access the brain.

19. Liver Transplant: Surgical replacement of a diseased liver with a healthy donor liver.

20. Kidney Transplant: Surgical transplantation of a healthy kidney into a recipient.

Surgical Instruments

21. Scalpel: A sharp knife used for surgical incisions.

22. Forceps: Tweezer-like instruments for grasping and holding tissues.

23. Hemostats: Clamps used to control bleeding from blood vessels.

24. Surgical Scissors: Scissors designed for cutting tissues.

25. Needle Holder: Instrument for holding and manipulating needles during suturing.

26. Sutures: Threads or stitches used to close incisions.

27. Retractors: Instruments used to hold back tissues to provide better visibility.

28. Electrocautery (Bovie): Device that uses electrical current to cut or coagulate tissues.

29. Trocar: A sharp-pointed instrument used for puncturing body cavities during laparoscopic procedures.

30. Surgical Drapes: Sterile coverings used to isolate the surgical area.

31. Speculum: An instrument used for opening and exposing body orifices.

32. Surgical Gown and Gloves: Sterile clothing for surgeons and surgical staff.

33. Suction Device: Used to remove fluids and debris during surgery.

34. Tourniquet: A device to temporarily stop blood flow to a limb during surgery.

35. Surgical Light: Illumination used to provide a well-lit surgical field.

36. Sterile Tray: A container for holding sterile instruments and supplies during surgery.

These terms describe various surgical procedures and instruments used by surgeons and medical professionals in surgical interventions and operations.

Medications and Pharmacology

Medical terms related to medications and pharmacology:

Medications

1. Antibiotics: Medications that treat bacterial infections.

2. Analgesics: Pain-relieving medications, including opioids and non-opioids.

3. Antipyretics: Medications that reduce fever.

4. Anti-inflammatories: Medications that reduce inflammation and pain.

5. Antidepressants: Medications used to treat depression and other mood disorders.

6. Antipsychotics: Medications for the treatment of psychotic disorders.

7. Antihypertensives: Medications that lower high blood pressure.

8. Diuretics: Medications that promote urine production and reduce fluid retention.

9. Anticoagulants: Medications that prevent blood clot formation.

10. Antihistamines: Medications that treat allergies and reduce histamine reactions.

11. Bronchodilators: Medications that open airways to treat respiratory conditions.

12. Immunosuppressants: Medications that suppress the immune system.

13. Antivirals: Medications that treat viral infections.

14. Antifungals: Medications that treat fungal infections.

15. Vaccines: Preparations to stimulate the immune system against specific diseases.

16. Steroids: Medications that reduce inflammation and suppress the immune system.

17. Anesthetics: Medications that induce temporary loss of sensation.

18. Hormone Replacement Therapy (HRT): Treatment to replace hormones in the body.

19. Opioid Reversal Agent (Naloxone): Medication to reverse opioid overdose.

20. Stimulants: Medications that increase alertness and energy.

21. Antiemetics: Medications that prevent or alleviate nausea and vomiting.

22. Muscle Relaxants: Medications that relax muscle tension.

23. Laxatives: Medications that promote bowel movements.

24. Antacids: Medications to neutralize stomach acid.

25. Antiplatelet Agents: Medications that prevent platelets from forming clots.
26. ACE Inhibitors: Medications that treat hypertension and heart conditions.

27. Statins: Medications to lower cholesterol levels.

28. Proton Pump Inhibitors (PPIs): Medications to reduce stomach acid production.

29. NSAIDs (Nonsteroidal Anti-Inflammatory Drugs): Medications that reduce pain and inflammation.

30. Beta-Blockers: Medications to treat heart conditions and hypertension.

31. Antiarrhythmics: Medications to control abnormal heart rhythms.

Pharmacology Terminology

32. Pharmacokinetics: The study of how the body absorbs, distributes, metabolizes, and excretes drugs.

33. Pharmacodynamics: The study of how drugs interact with the body to produce their effects.

34. Drug Interaction: The effect of one drug on the action of another drug.

35. Dose: The quantity of a medication administered at one time.

36. Route of Administration: The method by which a drug is introduced into the body (e.g., oral, intravenous).

37. Adverse Effects: Unintended and usually harmful effects of a medication.

38. Contraindications: Situations where a medication should not be used.

39. Tolerance: Reduced responsiveness to a drug over time.

40. Placebo: An inactive substance used in clinical trials for comparison.

41. Over-the-Counter (OTC): Medications available without a prescription.

42. Prescription Medication: Medications that require a healthcare provider's prescription.

These terms are essential in understanding the use, effects, and mechanisms of various medications and drugs in healthcare and pharmacology.

Therapeutic and Rehabilitative Procedures

Therapeutic Procedures

1. Physical Therapy (PT): A rehabilitative treatment that focuses on improving physical function, mobility, and pain management.

2. Occupational Therapy (OT): A therapy that helps individuals regain or develop daily life skills and functional independence.

3. Speech Therapy (Speech-Language Pathology): Treatment for communication disorders, speech, and language problems.

4. Counseling: Psychological therapy to address mental and emotional disorders and provide support.

5. Psychotherapy: Talk therapy that addresses emotional and psychological issues.

6. Radiation Therapy: The use of high-energy radiation to treat diseases, especially cancer.

7. Chemotherapy: The use of drugs to treat cancer and other diseases.

8. Electroconvulsive Therapy (ECT): A procedure that induces controlled seizures to treat mental illnesses.

9. Cardiac Rehabilitation: A program that helps patients recover from heart conditions through exercise and education.

10. Pulmonary Rehabilitation: A program to improve lung function and overall fitness in patients with respiratory conditions.

11. Wound Care: Treatment and management of wounds to promote healing.

12. Balneotherapy: Therapeutic use of mineral-rich water baths or spa treatments.

13. Hydrotherapy: Therapy involving the use of water for pain relief and physical rehabilitation.

14. Art Therapy: A form of expressive therapy using art to promote emotional healing.

15. Music Therapy: The use of music to improve mental and emotional well-being.

16. Massage Therapy: The manipulation of soft tissues to relieve pain and promote relaxation.

17. Occupational Rehabilitation: A program that helps individuals reenter the workforce after injury or illness.

Rehabilitative Procedures

18. Physical Rehabilitation: Comprehensive programs to improve physical function and mobility.

19. Vocational Rehabilitation: Assistance for individuals with disabilities to re-enter the workforce.

20. Orthopedic Rehabilitation: Rehabilitation for musculoskeletal injuries and surgeries.

21. Neurological Rehabilitation: Rehabilitation for individuals with neurological conditions, such as stroke or spinal cord injury.

22. Cardiac Rehabilitation: Programs for individuals recovering from heart-related conditions.

23. Speech and Language Rehabilitation: Programs to improve communication skills.

24. Cognitive Rehabilitation: Programs to address cognitive deficits due to brain injury or neurological conditions.

25. Substance Abuse Rehabilitation: Treatment for individuals with substance use disorders.

26. Amputee Rehabilitation: Rehabilitation for individuals who have had amputations.

27. Pediatric Rehabilitation: Rehabilitation programs tailored for children.

28. Geriatric Rehabilitation: Rehabilitation for elderly individuals, focusing on age-related conditions.

These terms cover a wide range of therapeutic and rehabilitative procedures and programs used to help individuals recover, regain function, and improve their well-being in various healthcare settings.

Chapter 5

Medical Specialties and Terminology

Medical Specialties

1. Cardiology: The branch of medicine that deals with the heart and circulatory system.

2. Dermatology: The study and treatment of skin disorders.

3. Gastroenterology: The field of medicine focused on the digestive system.

4. Neurology: The study and treatment of disorders of the nervous system.

5. Ophthalmology: The branch of medicine that specializes in eye care.

6. Orthopedics: The field that deals with the musculoskeletal system and orthopedic surgery.

7. Obstetrics and Gynecology (OB/GYN): Specialties dedicated to women's health and pregnancy.

8. Pediatrics: The medical care of infants, children, and adolescents.

9. Urology: The study and treatment of the urinary tract and male reproductive system.

10. Oncology: The field focused on the diagnosis and treatment of cancer.

11. Psychiatry: The branch of medicine that addresses mental health and mental disorders.

12. Radiology: The use of medical imaging techniques for diagnosis and treatment.

13. Nephrology: Specializes in kidney health and kidney disease treatment.

14. Endocrinology: The study of hormones and endocrine system disorders.

15. Pulmonology: Focuses on the respiratory system and lung diseases.

16. Rheumatology: The field of medicine dealing with autoimmune and musculoskeletal disorders.

17. Gynecologic Oncology: The study and treatment of gynecological cancers.

18. Anesthesiology: Specializes in providing anesthesia for surgical and medical procedures.

19. Emergency Medicine: The treatment of acute illnesses and injuries in the emergency department.

20. Infectious Disease: Specializes in the prevention, diagnosis, and treatment of infectious diseases.

21. Geriatrics: Focuses on the healthcare of elderly individuals.

22. Allergy and Immunology: The study and treatment of allergies and immune system disorders.

23. Hematology: Specializes in the study of blood and blood disorders.

24. Physical Medicine and Rehabilitation (PM&R): Focuses on physical therapy and rehabilitation.

25. Pathology: The study of the causes and effects of diseases.

26. Dentistry: The branch of medicine focused on oral health and dental care.

27. Nutrition and Dietetics: The science of food, nutrition, and diet.

28. Hospital Medicine: Specializes in the care of hospitalized patients.

29. Family Medicine: Offers comprehensive primary care for individuals and families.

30. Internal Medicine: Specializes in adult healthcare and complex medical conditions.

Medical Terminology

- Diagnosis: The identification of a disease or condition.

- Prognosis: The expected course and outcome of a disease.

- Symptom: A subjective indication of a disease or condition experienced by the patient.

- Sign: An objective, observable indication of a disease or condition.

- Treatment: The course of action taken to manage or cure a medical condition.

- Prescription: A written order for medication or treatment.

- Medical History: Information about a patient's past and present health.

- Patient Consultation: A meeting between a patient and a healthcare provider to discuss health concerns.

- Patient Records: Documents containing medical information and patient history.

- Medical Imaging: The use of various techniques to visualize internal body structures.

- Physical Examination: A visual and manual inspection of a patient's body.

- Laboratory Tests: Diagnostic tests performed on bodily fluids or tissues.

- Medication: A substance used to treat or prevent disease.

- Therapy: Treatment designed to alleviate or manage a health condition.

- Rehabilitation: A program to help patients regain function after injury or illness.

Specialized Fields in Medicine

These are some of them:

1. Cardiology: Specializes in the heart and circulatory system.

2. Dermatology: Focuses on skin disorders and dermatological conditions.

3. Gastroenterology: Specializes in the digestive system and gastrointestinal diseases.

4. Neurology: Deals with disorders of the nervous system.

5. Ophthalmology: Specializes in eye care, including vision and eye diseases.

6. Orthopedics: Concentrates on the musculoskeletal system, including bones and joints.

7. Obstetrics and Gynecology (OB/GYN): Devoted to women's health, pregnancy, and childbirth.

8. Pediatrics: Focuses on the healthcare of infants, children, and adolescents.

9. Urology: Specializes in the urinary tract and male reproductive system.

10. Oncology: Concerned with the diagnosis and treatment of cancer.

11. Psychiatry: Focuses on mental health and mental disorders.

12. Radiology: Uses medical imaging techniques for diagnosis and treatment.

13. Nephrology: Specializes in kidney health and kidney disease treatment.

14. Endocrinology: Studies hormones and endocrine system disorders.

15. Pulmonology: Concentrates on the respiratory system and lung diseases.

16. Rheumatology: Focuses on autoimmune and musculoskeletal disorders.

17. Gynecologic Oncology: Specializes in the study and treatment of gynecological cancers.

18. Anesthesiology: Specializes in providing anesthesia for surgical and medical procedures.

19. Emergency Medicine:Focuses on the treatment of acute illnesses and injuries in the emergency department.

20. Infectious Disease: Specializes in the prevention, diagnosis, and treatment of infectious diseases.

21. Geriatrics: Focuses on the healthcare of elderly individuals.

22. Allergy and Immunology: Specializes in the study and treatment of allergies and immune system disorders.

23. Hematology: Specializes in the study of blood and blood disorders.

24. Physical Medicine and Rehabilitation (PM&R): Focuses on physical therapy and rehabilitation.

25. Pathology: Studies the causes and effects of diseases.

26. Dentistry: Concentrates on oral health and dental care.

27. Nutrition and Dietetics: Involves the science of food, nutrition, and diet.

28. Hospital Medicine: Specializes in the care of hospitalized patients.

29. Family Medicine: Offers comprehensive primary care for individuals and families.

30. Internal Medicine: Specializes in adult healthcare and complex medical conditions.

These specialized fields in medicine cater to specific areas of healthcare and often require additional training and expertise in their respective domains.

Terminology for Healthcare Professionals

1. Patient Care: The provision of medical care, treatment, and support to patients.

2. Charting: The process of recording patient information and medical data.

3. Medical History: A patient's past and present health information.

4. Diagnosis: Identifying a patient's medical condition.

5. Prognosis: The expected course and outcome of a disease.

6. Symptom: A subjective indication of a disease or condition experienced by the patient.

7. Sign: An objective, observable indication of a disease or condition.

8. Treatment Plan: A plan outlining the course of action to manage or cure a patient's condition.

9. Medication: A substance used to treat or prevent disease.

10. Prescription: A written order for medication or treatment.

11. Informed Consent: Permission given by a patient to undergo a medical procedure or treatment after being informed of its risks and benefits.

12. HIPAA (Health Insurance Portability and Accountability Act):
A law protecting patient privacy and health information.

13. Medical Records: Documents containing a patient's medical history, treatment, and health information.

14. Medical Imaging: The use of various techniques to visualize internal body structures.

15. Physical Examination: A visual and manual inspection of a patient's body.

16. Vital Signs: Key physiological signs such as heart rate, blood pressure, and temperature.

17. Medical Chart: A visual representation of a patient's medical history.

18. CPR (Cardiopulmonary Resuscitation): Emergency life-saving procedure for cardiac and respiratory arrest.

19. Patient Consultation: A meeting between a patient and a healthcare provider to discuss health concerns.

20. EHR (Electronic Health Record): A digital record of a patient's health information.

21. ICD-10 (International Classification of Diseases, 10th Edition): A coding system used for billing and diagnosis.

22. SOAP Note (Subjective, Objective, Assessment, Plan): A structured format for medical notes.

23. Continuing Medical Education (CME): Ongoing education and training for healthcare professionals.

24. Telemedicine: The use of technology for remote patient care and consultations.

25. Medical Billing and Coding: The process of translating medical services into billing codes.

26. Malpractice: Professional negligence or misconduct by a healthcare provider.

27. Bioethics: The study of ethical issues in healthcare.

28. Medical Ethics: Ethical principles guiding medical practice.

29. DNR (Do Not Resuscitate): A patient's request not to receive CPR.

30. Morbidity: The state of being diseased.

31. Mortality: The state of being subject to death.

32. Healthcare Provider: A person or entity that delivers medical care.

33. Specialist: A healthcare professional who specializes in a specific area of medicine.

34. Residency: Postgraduate training for medical professionals.

35. JCAHO (Joint Commission on Accreditation of Healthcare Organizations): An organization that accredits healthcare institutions.

36. Malpractice Insurance: Insurance coverage for healthcare providers against liability.

37. PA (Physician Assistant): A healthcare professional who practices medicine under a licensed physician's supervision.

38. Nurse Practitioner: A registered nurse with advanced education and training.

39. Pharmacist: A healthcare professional who dispenses medications.

40. Medical School: A graduate institution for medical education.

These terms are essential for healthcare professionals to communicate, document, and provide effective patient care while adhering to ethical and legal standards.

These are the key terms related to medical records and documentation:

1. Electronic Health Record (EHR): A digital record of a patient's health information, including medical history, test results, and treatment plans.

2. Medical Chart: A visual representation of a patient's medical history, typically organized into sections for various types of information.

3. Patient Chart: A specific medical chart for an individual patient, containing their unique health information.

4. Charting: The process of recording and documenting patient information, such as symptoms, vital signs, and treatments.

5. Healthcare Documentation: The collection, organization, and storage of patient data for clinical, administrative, and legal purposes.

6. SOAP Note (Subjective, Objective, Assessment, Plan): A structured format for medical notes that includes information about the patient's condition, examination findings, assessment, and treatment plan.

7. Medical History: A comprehensive record of a patient's past and present health, including medical conditions, surgeries, allergies, and family history.

8. Diagnosis: The identification of a patient's medical condition based on clinical evaluation and test results.

9. Prognosis: The expected course and outcome of a disease or medical condition.

10. Medical Imaging Report: A written interpretation of medical imaging studies (e.g., X-rays, MRI, CT scans) by a radiologist.

11. Progress Notes: Ongoing documentation of a patient's condition, treatments, and progress during a hospital stay or outpatient care.

12. Vital Signs: Essential physiological measurements such as heart rate, blood pressure, temperature, and respiratory rate.

13. Informed Consent: Permission given by a patient to undergo a medical procedure or treatment after being informed of its risks and benefits.

14. HIPAA (Health Insurance Portability and Accountability Act): A law protecting patient privacy and the confidentiality of health information.

15. ICD-10 (International Classification of Diseases, 10th Edition): A coding system used for billing and diagnosis.

16. ICD-10-CM: A specific coding system used for clinical modification.

17. CPT (Current Procedural Terminology): Codes used for medical billing to describe medical procedures and services.

18. Health Information Management (HIM): The practice of managing health information throughout its lifecycle, including its collection, storage, analysis, and distribution.

19. JCAHO (Joint Commission on Accreditation of Healthcare Organizations): An organization that accredits healthcare institutions and sets standards for quality care.

20. Medical Coding: The process of translating medical services and diagnoses into alphanumeric codes for billing and insurance purposes.

21. Health Record Release Authorization: A patient's written consent to release their medical records to a specific party.

22. Telemedicine Documentation: Documentation of remote patient care and consultations conducted through technology.

23. Nurse's Notes: Documentation by nursing staff that includes observations, care provided, and patient interactions.

24. Operative Report: A surgeon's detailed documentation of a surgical procedure, including preoperative and postoperative details.

25. Physician's Orders: Written instructions from a physician regarding a patient's care, treatment, and medications.

Effective and accurate medical records and documentation are crucial for patient care, communication among healthcare professionals, legal compliance, and insurance billing.

Electronic Health Records (EHRs)

Related items to Electronic Health Records (EHRs):

1. Electronic Health Record (EHR): A digital version of a patient's paper medical chart, containing comprehensive health information, including medical history, diagnoses, medications, treatment plans, and more.

2. Health Information Exchange (HIE): The sharing of electronic health information among different healthcare organizations and systems to provide access to patient data across facilities and networks.

3. Patient Portal: An online platform that allows patients to access their EHR, schedule appointments, communicate with healthcare providers, and view test results.

4. Meaningful Use: A set of standards and criteria established by the Centers for Medicare & Medicaid Services (CMS) to encourage the adoption and meaningful use of EHRs.

5. Interoperability: The ability of EHR systems to communicate and share patient data with other EHR systems and healthcare entities.

6. Personal Health Record (PHR): An electronic record maintained by the patient, containing their health information, allowing them to manage and share their medical data.

7. Health Information Technology (HIT): The use of technology to store, manage, and exchange health information, including EHRs and related systems.

8. EHR Integration: The process of incorporating EHR systems with other healthcare applications and technologies, such as lab systems or pharmacy systems.

9. Data Migration: The transfer of patient data from paper records or one EHR system to another.

10. EHR Vendor: A company that develops, sells, and supports EHR software and systems for healthcare organizations.

11. Clinical Decision Support (CDS): Software tools that assist healthcare providers in making clinical decisions by providing patient-specific information and treatment recommendations.

12. Electronic Prescribing (e-Prescribing): The digital process of sending prescriptions directly to pharmacies from EHR systems.

13. Health Information Management (HIM):The practice of managing health information, including the collection, storage, analysis, and distribution of patient data within EHRs.

14. Telehealth: The use of technology to provide remote medical care and consultations, often integrated with EHRs.

15. EHR Training: Education and training for healthcare professionals and staff to effectively use EHR systems.

16. Healthcare Analytics: The use of data from EHRs and other sources to analyze and improve patient care, outcomes, and operational efficiency.

17. EHR Certification: A process by which EHR systems are tested and certified to meet certain standards and criteria, ensuring they are capable of supporting meaningful use.

18. HL7 (Health Level Seven): A set of international standards for the exchange, integration, sharing, and retrieval of electronic health information.

19. Audit Trail: A record of who accessed, modified, or viewed patient data within an EHR system, providing transparency and security.

20. EHR Workflow: The sequence of steps and processes for inputting, managing, and retrieving electronic health information.

EHRs have revolutionized healthcare by providing a more efficient and accessible way to manage patient data, improve patient care, and streamline healthcare processes.

Proper Documentation and Terminology

Proper documentation and terminology are crucial in healthcare to ensure accurate communication, patient safety, and legal compliance, key aspects:

1. Accuracy: Document information accurately, including patient details, medical history, symptoms, vital signs, and diagnoses. Use standardized terminology to eliminate ambiguity.

2. Consistency: Maintain consistency in documenting patient data to enable easy retrieval and understanding by other healthcare professionals.

3. Clarity: Use clear and concise language to convey information. Avoid jargon or abbreviations that may be unclear to others.

4. Privacy and Confidentiality: Safeguard patient privacy and comply with HIPAA regulations. Limit access to sensitive data and ensure it's securely stored.

5. Timeliness: Document patient information promptly after interactions to prevent errors or omissions.

6. Standardized Terminology: Use standardized medical terminology and coding systems like ICD-10, CPT, and SNOMED CT to ensure accurate communication and billing.

7. SOAP Notes: Utilize the SOAP note format (Subjective, Objective, Assessment, Plan) to structure documentation, making it organized and easily understandable.

8. Consents and Authorizations: Properly document informed consent for treatments and procedures, ensuring that patients understand the risks and benefits.

9. Data Integrity: Maintain the integrity of electronic health records (EHRs) by preventing unauthorized alterations and maintaining an audit trail.

10. Risk Management: Document any patient incidents or adverse events thoroughly and in a timely manner for risk management and legal purposes.

11. Medication Documentation: Clearly document medication names, dosages, routes, and administration times. Avoid medication errors through accurate recording.

12. Allergies and Adverse Reactions: Document patient allergies and adverse reactions to medications or treatments to prevent potential harm.

13. Communication: Ensure that documentation facilitates effective communication among healthcare team members, allowing them to provide optimal care.

14. Patient Education: Document patient education, including explanations of diagnoses, treatment options, and post-care instructions.

15. Signature and Credentials: Sign and date all entries in patient records with your professional credentials to authenticate your documentation.

16. Legal Requirements: Understand and adhere to legal and regulatory requirements for documentation in your jurisdiction, such as state and federal laws.

17. Avoid Copy-Pasting: Minimize the use of copy-pasting in EHRs to maintain the accuracy and relevance of information.

18. Correction of Errors: If errors are made, follow institutional protocols for correcting documentation, including clearly indicating the correction.

Proper documentation and standardized terminology are essential to provide quality patient care, facilitate communication, and meet legal and regulatory standards in healthcare. They help ensure that patients receive accurate, safe, and effective medical treatment.

Case studies and practice are valuable tools in healthcare education and professional development. They offer real-world scenarios that allow healthcare professionals to apply their knowledge and skills. Here are some key points related to case studies and practice in healthcare:

Case Studies

1. Definition: Case studies are detailed, in-depth examinations of specific patient cases or medical scenarios. They often include patient history, clinical findings, test results, and the course of treatment.

2. Educational Tool: Case studies are used in medical schools, nursing programs, and continuing education to teach students and professionals how to diagnose and treat medical conditions.

3. Problem-Solving: They encourage critical thinking and problem-solving by requiring individuals to analyze complex clinical situations and make informed decisions.

4. Interdisciplinary Learning: Case studies often involve collaboration among healthcare professionals from various disciplines, such as doctors, nurses, and pharmacists.

5. Realistic Scenarios: They provide a bridge between theoretical knowledge and real-world application, helping learners understand the complexities of patient care.

Practice in Healthcare

1. Clinical Practice: Healthcare professionals apply their knowledge and skills in real patient care settings, including hospitals, clinics, and other healthcare facilities.

2. Simulation Training: Healthcare simulation is a form of practice that allows learners to work with mannequins, virtual patients, or standardized patients to practice clinical skills and scenarios in a safe environment.

3. Continuing Education: Practicing healthcare professionals engage in ongoing training and practice to stay current with advancements in their field.

4. Competency Assessment: Healthcare institutions use practice to assess the competency of their staff and ensure they can perform clinical tasks safely and effectively.

5. Skills Refinement: Regular practice helps healthcare professionals refine their clinical skills and maintain a high level of expertise.

6. Teamwork and Communication: Interprofessional practice encourages collaboration and effective communication among healthcare team members to ensure optimal patient care.

7. Patient Safety: Practice contributes to improved patient safety by reducing medical errors and enhancing the quality of care.

8. Evidence-Based Practice: Healthcare professionals rely on current research and evidence to guide their clinical practice and decision-making.

Case studies and practice are fundamental in the development and enhancement of clinical skills, diagnostic abilities, and decision-making in healthcare. They bridge the gap between theory and real-world patient care, ultimately benefiting both healthcare professionals and the patients they serve.

Self-Assessment Exercises

Self-assessment exercises that healthcare professionals can use to evaluate and improve their skills and knowledge:

1. Clinical Knowledge Quiz: Take quizzes or tests related to your field to assess your clinical knowledge.

2. Case Study Analysis: Analyze patient case studies, make diagnoses, and create treatment plans to enhance your clinical decision-making.

3. Clinical Skills Checklist: Use a checklist to evaluate and rate your proficiency in various clinical skills.

4. Peer Review: Collaborate with colleagues to review and provide feedback on each other's clinical practices.

5. Simulation Scenarios: Engage in simulated patient scenarios to practice clinical skills and decision-making.

6. Ethical Dilemma Analysis: Reflect on and assess your handling of ethical dilemmas and complex moral situations in healthcare.

7. Evidence-Based Practice Review: Evaluate your adherence to evidence-based guidelines and practices in your field.

8. Patient Communication Assessment: Assess your patient communication skills, including active listening, empathy, and clear explanations.

9. Time Management Evaluation: Review your ability to manage time effectively in a clinical setting to ensure efficient patient care.

10. Conflict Resolution Practice: Practice managing conflicts and challenging interactions with patients, families, or colleagues.

11. Cultural Competency Self-Assessment: Reflect on your cultural competence and how you provide culturally sensitive care.

12. Leadership Skills Evaluation: Assess your leadership skills and effectiveness in interprofessional teamwork.

13. Stress Management Assessment: Regularly evaluate your stress management strategies and mental well-being to provide effective care.

14. Clinical Documentation Review: Examine your medical record-keeping to ensure accuracy, completeness, and compliance with standards.

15. Professional Development Plan: Create a personalized development plan with goals, areas for improvement, and strategies for growth.

16. Patient Experience Feedback: Seek feedback from patients about their experiences with your care and communication.

17. Interprofessional Collaboration Assessment: Evaluate your ability to work effectively in healthcare teams and communicate with other professionals.

18. Continuing Education Assessment: Monitor your participation in and completion of continuing education courses to stay current in your field.

19. Clinical Competency Exams: Take clinical competency exams or assessments specific to your area of expertise.

20. Quality Improvement Initiatives: Participate in quality improvement projects and assess your contributions to enhancing patient care.

These self-assessment exercises help healthcare professionals identify areas for improvement, maintain competence, and provide high-quality patient care. They can be adapted to fit your specific field and professional goals.

Applying Medical Terminology in Case Studies

Applying medical terminology in case studies is a valuable exercise for healthcare professionals, students, and educators. It allows individuals to integrate their knowledge of medical language into practical clinical scenarios.This is how you can apply medical terminology in case studies:

1. Case Selection: Choose a case study that aligns with the medical specialty or topic you want to focus on. Ensure that the case is comprehensive and includes patient history, symptoms, clinical findings, diagnoses, and treatment plans.

2. Analyze Patient Data: Review the case study and identify medical terms and phrases relevant to the patient's condition. This includes medical history, symptoms, physical examination findings, diagnostic tests, and treatment modalities.

3. Use Medical Terminology: Apply appropriate medical terminology to describe and document the patient's condition. Use accurate anatomical and physiological terms to specify the location and nature of any abnormalities.

4. Diagnosis: Utilize medical terminology to diagnose the patient's condition. This may involve recognizing diagnostic codes (e.g., ICD-10) that correspond to the identified medical conditions.

5. Treatment Plan: Describe the treatment plan using medical terminology. Include details about medications, surgical procedures, therapies, and any other interventions.

6. Documentation: Practice creating SOAP notes (Subjective, Objective, Assessment, Plan) using medical terminology. Ensure that your notes are concise, accurate, and organized.

7. Interpret Test Results: Interpret diagnostic test results in the case study, explaining abnormal findings in medical terms and linking them to the diagnosis.

8. Medical Abbreviations: Use appropriate medical abbreviations but ensure that you expand them or provide their meanings when they are first introduced in the case study.

9. Communication: If the case study involves interactions with other healthcare professionals or patients, use appropriate medical terminology to communicate effectively.

10. Apply Critical Thinking: Utilize critical thinking skills to determine the most suitable medical terminology for the case, considering context and relevance.

11. Reflect and Discuss: After analyzing the case study, reflect on your findings, discuss them with peers or instructors, and seek feedback to improve your application of medical terminology.

12. Continual Practice: Regularly work with case studies that cover various medical specialties to enhance your proficiency in using medical terminology in different contexts.

By applying medical terminology in case studies, healthcare professionals and students can reinforce their understanding of medical language and its practical applications in clinical settings. This exercise contributes to improved patient care, accurate documentation, and effective communication within the healthcare team.

These are some of the common medical abbreviations:

1. Rx: Prescription

2. Dx: Diagnosis

3. Tx : Treatment

4. Hx : Medical history

5. CC: Chief Complaint

6. CXR: Chest X-ray

7. ECG or EKG: Electrocardiogram

8. MRI: Magnetic Resonance Imaging

9. CT: Computed Tomography

10. BP: Blood Pressure

11. HR: Heart Rate

12. RR: Respiratory Rate
13. TPR: Temperature, Pulse, Respiration

14. CBC: Complete Blood Count

15. WBC: White Blood Cell

16. RBC: Red Blood Cell

17. ESR: Erythrocyte
Sedimentation Rate

18. IV: Intravenous

19. PO: By mouth (oral)

20. NPO: Nothing by mouth (nothing per oral)

21. PRN: As needed (pro re nata)

22. QD: Once a day (every day)

23. BID: Twice a day (two times a day)

24. TID: Three times a day (three times a day

25. QID: Four times a day (four times a day)

26. QHS: Every night at bedtime

27. NKA: No Known Allergies

28. SOB: Shortness of Breath

29. GI: Gastrointestinal

30. GU: Genitourinary

31. CVA: Cerebrovascular Accident (Stroke)

32. MI: Myocardial Infarction (Heart Attack)

33. COPD: Chronic Obstructive Pulmonary Disease

34. GERD: Gastroesophageal Reflux Disease

35. DM: Diabetes Mellitus

36. HTN: Hypertension (High Blood Pressure)

37. CA: Cancer

38. MMS: Multiple Sclerosis

39. HIV: Human Immunodeficiency Virus

40. AIDS: Acquired Immunodeficiency Syndrome

41. UTI: Urinary Tract Infection

42. OB/GYN: Obstetrics and Gynecology

43. ENT: Ear, Nose, and Throat

44. ASAP: As Soon As Possible

45. N/V: Nausea and Vomiting

46. CABG: Coronary Artery Bypass Graft

47. CHF: Congestive Heart Failure

48. SIRS: Systemic Inflammatory Response Syndrome

49. PT: Physical Therapy

50. OT: Occupational Therapy

51. ROM: Range of Motion

52. POA: Power of Attorney

53. DOA: Dead on Arrival

54. NPO: Nil per os (Nothing by mouth)

55. DC: Discharge

56. ROS: Review of Systems

57. LOC: Loss of Consciousness

58. Fx: Fracture

59. VS: Vital Signs

60. DNR: Do Not Resuscitate

61. ICU: Intensive Care Unit

62. ER: Emergency Room

63. NICU: Neonatal Intensive Care Unit

64. OB: Obstetrics

65. PPD: Purified Protein Derivative (Tuberculosis skin test)

66. DVT: Deep Vein Thrombosis

67. ABG: Arterial Blood Gas

68. CPR: Cardiopulmonary Resuscitation

69. APAP: Acetaminophen (Paracetamol)

70. GER: Gastroesophageal Reflux

71. PPI: Proton Pump Inhibitor

72. DMARD: Disease-Modifying Antirheumatic Drug

73. TSH: Thyroid-Stimulating Hormone

74. ICD: International Classification of Diseases

75. MRI: Magnetic
Resonance Imaging

76. TPA: Tissue Plasminogen Activator

77. IVF: In Vitro Fertilization

78. ENT: Ear, Nose, and Throat

79. PID: Pelvic Inflammatory

80. ARDS: Acute Respiratory Distress Syndrome

Please note that this list includes a variety of medical abbreviations commonly used in healthcare and medical documentation.